Fighting Glaucoma
An Action Handbook

DISCLAIMER

While all reasonable efforts have been made to supply complete and accurate information and to ensure that the methodologies presented in this book function as described, the authors and publisher offer this publication without warranty of any kind and accept no responsibility for its use.

Fighting Glaucoma
An Action Handbook

Ivan Goldberg
Nahum Goldmann

First edition

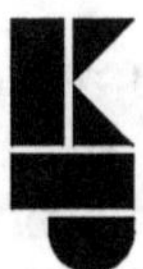

Kugler Publications/Amsterdam/The Netherlands

ISBN 978-90-6299-311-6

Standard soft cover print-on-demand edition. See our website for premium editions of our books.

Kugler Publications
P.O. Box 20538
1001 NM Amsterdam, The Netherlands
www.kuglerpublications.com

Kugler Publications is an imprint of SPB Academic Publishing bv, P.O. Box 20538, 1001 NM Amsterdam, The Netherlands

Cover design: Willem Driebergen, Rijnsburg, The Netherlands

Cover photo by Paul Morris on Unsplash (www.unsplash.com)

Authors dedicate this book to all their relatives, friends and the professionals, who do care; and who were kind enough to help, when we inevitably required compassion and help.

Table of contents

Acknowledgments

In this book, we draw on the academic knowledge and practical experience of many glaucoma researchers and medical practitioners, to whom we are especially indebted.

We are also thankful to those publishers and authors who gave us permission to quote their publications.

Most importantly, I, Ivan Goldberg, am indebted to Vera and our children and grandchildren for inspiring and continuously grounding me, along with my many patients who continue to teach me daily.

Nahum Goldmann is happy to acknowledge Natalya, Alice, Naomi-Roni, Mirele-Bella and Marat for their constant inspiration, support, encouragement and love.

Foreword

Glaucoma affects over 60 million people worldwide and is the leading cause of irreversible blindness. At least half of those affected do not know that they have it. Those who do, are often frustrated in their search for valid and trustworthy information about their disease (there are many different forms of glaucoma) and what they should understand about its nature and treatment in order to obtain the best outcome.

For best results from treatment for glaucoma, patients need to be actively involved in the planning and carrying out of their own care. To be able to do this, they need to understand what is at stake, what needs to be done to save their sight, to know what to do and how to do it. While most of this knowledge comes from a strong relationship with a caring ophthalmologist, a great deal more could be gained with the help of a reader-friendly book that reinforces that knowledge and understanding.

There is a great deal of information, and also misinformation, on the internet, and many advertisements for treatments which may be not yet tested and proven, such as stem cell treatment. Over the years, there have been several books written for patients about glaucoma. What is needed, however, is a book that is written understandably, honestly, and fully explanatory of the different aspects of the nature, causation, manifestations, and treatment of glaucoma, plus information to guide the reader in searching for further information and assistance.

The book *Glaucoma: How to Save Your Sight* written by Professors Goldberg and Susanna does just that, and now this companion book by Professors Goldberg and Goldmann augments it effectively. This is a work produced by two extremely well-known, talented and knowledgeable authors and the two manuals should be in the possession of all glaucoma patients, and their ophthalmologists as well.

Robert Ritch, MD, FACS

Shelley and Steven Einhorn Distinguished Chair
 Professor of Ophthalmology
Surgeon Director Emeritus and Chief, Glaucoma Services
The New York Eye and Ear Infirmary of Mount Sinai
310 East 14th Street, New York, NY 10003, USA

Introduction

Most likely, gentle reader, you would rather have not opened a book with such a title, unless you felt driven to do so. Probably, you are reading it because you – or someone close to you – has been diagnosed with glaucoma and is on treatment. You might feel that you or this cherished someone might be on the road to losing sight, whether partially or fully; a scary possibility.

As written in the recent book by Professors I. Goldberg and R. Susanna Jr., which we extensively cite in this handbook:

"Glaucoma is infamous as 'the sneak thief of sight': the most common types give no warning. They are slowly, progressively destroying a person's vision. Because usually the vision at first is affected to the side, patients notice little, if anything. By the time an individual realizes something is wrong, there may have been considerable damage.

… Losing vision from glaucoma is tragic. It should be avoidable for most, but unfortunately not all, patients. When it occurs, as in most air crashes, this disaster may follow a combination of misperceptions and oversights, each contributing differently to the final result. Sometimes the disease is relentless no matter what is done; sometimes it deceives the clinician as much as the patient."

Glaucoma: At times, it is about hard choices

You might need to make some difficult choices, taking on commitments and responsibilities that are likely to apply for the rest of your life. With this book, we wish to help you to make these choices with as much relevant information as you might need. We want to help you to find the inner strength to fight this disease successfully. In a long journey, support from your family and friends will be invaluable.

Regrettably, glaucoma currently remains incurable. Owing to the injury it causes to the optic nerves in one or both of your eyes, any damage to your vision, which would have been quite unexpected, cannot be reversed. The good news is that most often, glaucoma can be controlled; that is, certain treatments could help to prevent blindness or, at least, to slow down any further decline in your vision.

New medical research results, testing and treatment methods become available daily, although progress towards a glaucoma cure is not as rapid as we would like it to be. Even if today for glaucoma patients fully preserving steady vision is not a certainty, your chances for stability might be quite reasonable – providing you make informed choices and take good care of your eyes by following the treatments prescribed by your caring physicians.

Because you are reading our handbook, we understand and respect that retaining as much vision as possible, for as long as you live, has become a major goal for you.

We, the authors

This handbook has been written by an unlikely combination of a physician and a patient. We live on opposite sides of the world, and collaborate through the internet. Our educations, experiences, viewpoints and motivations for writing this book are quite different.

Ivan Goldberg is a world-recognized expert in glaucoma treatment, on which subject he has published hundreds of articles, book chapters and a book and has been honored with numerous international awards. He is Head of the Glaucoma Unit, Sydney Eye Hospital, Director of Eye Associates, Sydney, Australia, and Clinical Professor at the University of Sydney. Dr. Goldberg was also President of the Royal Australian and New Zealand College of Ophthalmologists, President of the World Glaucoma Association, Foundation President of the Asia Pacific Glaucoma Society, Chair of the Australian and New Zealand Glaucoma Society and President of Glaucoma Australia. He has been an executive or honorary member of many Ophthalmology and Glaucoma research societies globally. Ivan Goldberg's most recent book is *Glaucoma: How to save your sight!* (co-authored with Prof. R. Susanna Jr., University of Sao Paulo, Brazil). It is an example of his abiding interest in the patient's perspective in glaucoma management, patient-related outcomes of treatment and a patient's quality of life.

Nahum Goldmann is an experienced high-tech executive, university professor and information scientist, with the considerable background in biophysics, biomedicine and health related subjects, who resides in Canada. Nahum's most recent book is *Effective Decision Making: A Primer in Information Retrieval*.

What united us in writing this book is a desire to help people with glaucoma in a practical way. We trust the differences we bring to this venture will enhance the usefulness of this handbook for you.

For a qualified medical practitioner, providing help usually means concentrating on better and clinically proven ways to treat the disease. In contrast, the long-term challenges faced by people with glaucoma are numerous and important. With such a diagnosis, you have to balance many life demands, of which eye treatments are essential but by no means alone.

After all, you are not living to treat glaucoma: you are living a full life into which the treatment of your condition is an intrusion. How could one cope?

Treatment of any chronic and serious medical condition is likely to be affected by many other factors, such as money, the wellbeing of your family, your general health, other calls on your time, fitness and lifestyle, housing, your work commitments, and perhaps supporting family members, to name just a few.

Our experience is complementary; we hope this builds a common and inclusive perspective for your benefit.

About this book... and a couple of others

Several books written for patients describe what glaucoma is, how it is being treated, and the state of glaucoma research. We are unaware of a book on *how to live with the glaucomas*, covering practical challenges frequently faced by those with glaucoma, who wish to minimize risk of visual disability or even blindness. We hope our book at least partly fills this void.

We try to address specific issues and anxieties that people with glaucoma might face daily, whether large or small. We aim to guide newly diagnosed individuals, their family and friends, on 'what is best to do' – and 'why'. We have seen such 'what to do' questions repeatedly on various glaucoma blogs.

This handbook's focus is on the step-by-step actions that you, as well as supporting relatives and friends, can take to improve your current situation and outlook. We try to guide you where to find additional help to understand better your condition and your prospects. We hope health professionals who help people with glaucoma also find this book useful.

We try to minimize information intake while maximizing personal actions available. We do not explain in much detail various types of glaucoma or cite references to scientific sources, unless it is necessary to validate recommended action. In such cases, we try to present relevant science pragmatically, without specialized medical jargon. With some exceptions, we also minimize formal citations to scientific sources.

You could use this handbook as an everyday reference or as a guide to your glaucoma treatment. We hope you will find it worthwhile to formulate better the reasons for your actions and for your sometimes complicated choices.

To those who would like to learn more about the glaucomas with background science, we recommend a companion book by one of our co-authors, *Glaucoma: How to save your sight!*, by I. Goldberg and R. Susanna Jr. (Kugler Publications, 2015). This book, which we extensively cite below as '*Goldberg/Susanna*', covers glaucoma research and medical practices in lay terms, with many details and numerous illustrations.

Perhaps you still do not feel that you have enough information to make an informed choice for your treatment, do not know how to get it, or would just like to dig more deeply into specialized medical literature, to identify and track more recent glaucoma research and treatments publications. Then, you might benefit from a book by our other co-author, *Effective Decision Making: A Primer in Information Retrieval*, 3rd Edition, by Nahum Goldmann, ARRAY Development, 2016. That book explains how to conduct effective online searching of scientific and biomedical literature.

A digital version of this handbook could be read using computerized gadgets for visually impaired. It could also be computer-translated on the fly to various other languages and without cost, thus reaching the worldwide majority of glaucoma patients who do not read English. *See information in the Appendix below on how you can find an appropriate computerized reading device or translate our handbook to the language of your choice.*

Request for additional questions

We envision this handbook as an evergreen source of common sense answers to your frequently asked questions. To achieve this, our readers, interested patients and eye health practitioners could submit to us questions about and practical solutions for glaucoma-induced challenges.

Chapter 1. Coming to terms: First steps

In this chapter, we discuss first steps you might take to confirm and clarify the initial diagnosis.

For many people, when they hear that they have glaucoma, the news comes as an unexpected shock. Even if they have heard this term before, not many know what it actually means. Many think of blindness; some might confuse glaucoma with other eye disorders, like cataracts or trachoma.

Eye health professionals, caregivers, relatives and friends could provide you with precious physical and psychological support, especially if they have the knowledge contained in this handbook. As glaucoma is a chronic and potentially debilitating disease without a known cure, you should spare no effort to ensure your doctor-patient relationship works for you. First and foremost, your vision is your responsibility.

If you are a child or sibling of a glaucoma patient

According to the research noted in *Goldberg/Susanna*, if one of your first-degree relatives (parent or sibling) has been diagnosed with glaucoma, your chances to get it jump tenfold! As well:

"Glaucomas are also more common in individuals who suffer from migraine, cold hands and feet in winter, diabetes, short-sightedness, high or conversely low blood pressure, those who smoke and those who have had to use steroid-type medications for long periods."

Overall, glaucoma affects about 2% of people over 40 years of age and increases with age, so that one person in 200 has glaucoma at the age of 40, while 8% of 80-year-olds have it; it is not that rare to start with. However, citing averages often misleads by concealing that for certain ethnic groups, sex, types of glaucoma and individual human traits, the genetically predisposed likelihood of getting glaucoma might be higher or lower.

As an example, just 0.75% of European-ethnicity men between the ages of 40 and 79 are estimated to develop glaucoma with an identifiable cause, exfoliation syndrome. For certain subgroups of the Ashkenazi Jews, the comparable probability of developing exfoliative glaucoma is three times higher at 2.2%.

The earlier glaucoma is diagnosed, the less damage it has had time to cause. However, according to *Goldberg/ Susanna*:

*"Even in developed societies, about 50% of patients with glaucoma have not been diagnosed and are not on treatment. **Half of these undiagnosed people have been seen by an eye health care practitioner in the last two years.** In developing nations the proportion of glaucoma sufferers undiagnosed may be well over 90% (especially in rural environments). When many of these undiagnosed patients are finally discovered, tragically, the glaucoma is often advanced.*

... It is only when the damage is sufficiently extensive for the brain to make mistakes that we start to fall over things, trip on stairs we did not see, knock into people on the side we did not know were there. This has huge implications for safe mobility, independent living and working as well as driving.

… It is the side vision that is destroyed in glaucoma, which for the reasons above, you do not miss until it is advanced. The vision used to read, write, recognize faces, watch TV, which would be missed immediately if it were to be damaged, is spared until late in glaucoma.

… You cannot reliably judge yourself how much damage this sneaky disease has caused to your sight, or tell accurately whether that damage is stable (treatment is protecting you) or getting worse."

If your parent or sibling has been diagnosed with glaucoma or you have other risk factors as listed above, like diabetes or cold hands and feet in winter, or if your eye pressure (intraocular pressure or IOP) is unusually high, you should consider the following key steps:

- If your age is 35 years or older, *schedule your own second yearly eye examinations by an ophthalmologist or an optometrist*, and ensure that the examination includes not only measuring your IOP but also, critically, a check of your optic nerves by a qualified person.

- As corneal central thickness was found to be an independent risk factor in progression from ocular hypertension to early glaucoma, ask your ophthalmologist whether ultrasonic pachymetry should be performed on your eyes to establish your baseline corneal thickness.

- Notify your doctors if you are planning a baby, are already expecting, or are breastfeeding, as this will strongly influence the safe treatment choices available to you, should you need eye drops.

- Babies with eyes that are too big or with one side bigger than the other, might have congenital glaucoma. Other warning signs include watering eyes and abnormal sensitivity to light. This rare kind of glaucoma affects about one baby in 10,000 births.

- Arrange genetic tests to identify at least in part your personal risk of glaucoma and, as a priceless gift to your children and grandchildren, of other contributing health risks or genetic predispositions that you or they might have. *Discuss in confidence your test results with your trusted genetic advisor or medical practitioner. See information in the Appendix below on how you can find an appropriate genetic testing service that could determine your personal chances of getting glaucoma and of many other potential health risks.*

- In cases when you have a predisposition to a secondary glaucoma, such as exfoliation syndrome, *discuss this increased risk with your doctor: in some situations, you might be able to take steps to prevent it.*

- Become aware of your local or a credible international glaucoma patient association or research foundation and support their efforts to spread glaucoma information and to advance glaucoma treatments. Remember, with the glaucoma present in your family, this is a good investment not just in your own health but also into the future for your children and grandchildren. *See information in the Appendix below on how you can contact your country's ophthalmology society or medical association that could put you in touch with the glaucoma researchers of your choice.*

On its own, raised IOP does not necessarily mean you have glaucoma, but the higher the IOP the greater the risk. Reducing IOP often slows further damage to the optic nerves that link the eye to the brain and convey the messages of sight.

Some people believe that if their IOP is less than 21 mmHg, they could not have glaucoma. However, according to *Goldberg/Susanna*:

> *"... 30% of Caucasians, 80% of Koreans and 90% of Japanese with glaucoma have never had elevated IOP measured. This makes diagnosis more challenging and may lead to glaucoma being missed, with possibly nasty results.*

> *... Eye pressure is a major risk factor for glaucoma: the higher it is, the greater the risk.* ***But eye pressure levels are NOT synonymous with a glaucoma diagnosis.*** *Not for many years has 'increased' IOP been part of the definition of glaucoma."*

One cannot really do anything specific to 'prevent' glaucoma before it develops (other than treat eye angle closure if your ophthalmologist were concerned about it). For you, planning eye care essentially means periodically evaluating your individual risks to determine the best and safest health strategy. In addition to the annual monitoring of IOP, this might even include initiation of IOP lowering treatment at the recommendation of your doctor.

A special concern for babies might be glaucoma associated with facial 'port wine stain' or 'birth mark'. If a person is born with this condition, it means the pressure in the veins behind and around the eye could be elevated, which could lead to a raised eye pressure. If the upper eyelid is involved in the stain, the risk of this kind of glaucoma is about 50%. Early treatment offers protection from visual damage, while a neurological assessment is also required.

You and your siblings and children should also pay attention to the many general factors that should be optimized for your overall health, such as ensuring normal blood pressure (not too high and not too low, including at night while you are sleeping), controlling high cholesterol and diabetes, detecting and treating sleep apnea. For a more detailed discussion of these issues, refer to the Goldberg/ Susanna book.

Substantiating your diagnosis

If you just have been told you have glaucoma, ensure this diagnosis has been made by a qualified ophthalmologist. If not, you might need to substantiate the diagnosis.

All physicians and allied eye care professionals are human; despite best efforts, anyone could make mistakes. A majority of people in the world live far from well-established medical centers, where local health professionals might not have specialized glaucoma training and access to modern diagnostic equipment or where qualified ophthalmologists are rare, and their diagnosis could not be independently confirmed with a second opinion.

Poor communication and inadequate documentation could happen even at the best medical institutions. Hence, inaccurate diagnosis might take place even under the best of circumstances.

- If you cannot easily find in your city or your country a qualified ophthalmologist, consider searching for an eye specialist in a nearby country or in a country with a similar linguistic or cultural profile. *Using information in the Appendix below, identify your target country's ophthalmology society or medical association that could put you in touch with a reputable ophthalmologist.*

- Alternatively, you might consider certain countries whose medical clinics have good reputations for treating foreign patients. Countries like Australia, Canada, most of the European Union, India, Ireland, Israel, Japan, Korea, New Zealand, Singapore, UK and USA are well regarded around the globe for the high quality of their medical treatment centers. *See information in the Appendix below on how you can contact your target country's trade representative, who could put you in touch with their country's leading medical clinics specializing in treating eye diseases.*

- If you have any reason to doubt the diagnosis given to you, *it is your right and responsibility to obtain a qualified second opinion.* This could be done by identifying a specialized ophthalmology clinic in your city or your country. *See information in the Appendix below on how you can contact your country's ophthalmology society or medical association that could put you in touch with an alternative ophthalmologist.*

Glaucoma origins and initial evaluation

Glaucoma is a group of eye diseases, all somewhat different in their physiological origins. Common to all glaucomas is damage to the optic nerve, which leads to irreversible sight loss.

Each eye's optic nerve consists at birth of about 1,200,000 very small nerve fibers that carry the messages of sight from your eye to brain. Once a particular nerve fiber dies, it cannot regenerate on its own. The more of these nerve fibers that die, the more severe your sight loss.

Optic nerve cell damage often follows high pressures inside your eyes, but also might occur at usual eye pressures for your ethnic group and age. Any rise in eye pressure is typically caused by the poor functioning of the circular mesh-like 'drain', overall smaller than 0.5 mm, which channels flow out of your eye of the clear watery 'aqueous' fluid, necessary for eye functioning and health.

In another kind of glaucoma, there might be crowding of this drain: as we age, the focusing lens of the eye just behind the drain channel slowly grows, thereby crowding the approach to the channel. If your drain channel is inherently narrow, this might become worse with time. When such narrowing reaches a critical level, the outflow drain can become blocked slowly or quickly, and eye pressure can buildup and damage the optic nerves.

As noted in *Goldberg/Susanna*:

> *"Effective treatment depends on an accurate diagnosis and this is entirely the ophthalmologist's responsibility."*

Your ophthalmologist uses a bio-microscope (slit lamp) to examine your eye under high magnification; to assess whether the cul-de-sac at the edge of the front chamber of the eye (from where the watery fluid drains out of your eye – the drainage angle) is open wide, or open but narrow, or closed; and to find any scarring or other damage to the drainage angle. During this brief test, the slit lamp light is directed at the drainage angle through a special mirror lens.

Your eyes are anesthetized with drops, so the test is painless for you.

Clarifying your diagnosis

Examination by your eye doctor aims to diagnose not only whether or not there is glaucoma present, but if so, what type of glaucoma you have and what damage it has caused up to that point in time. This influences treatment strategies. If at the time of initial diagnosis, glaucoma has caused advanced damage, early or even rarely immediate surgery might be necessary to reduce IOP adequately.

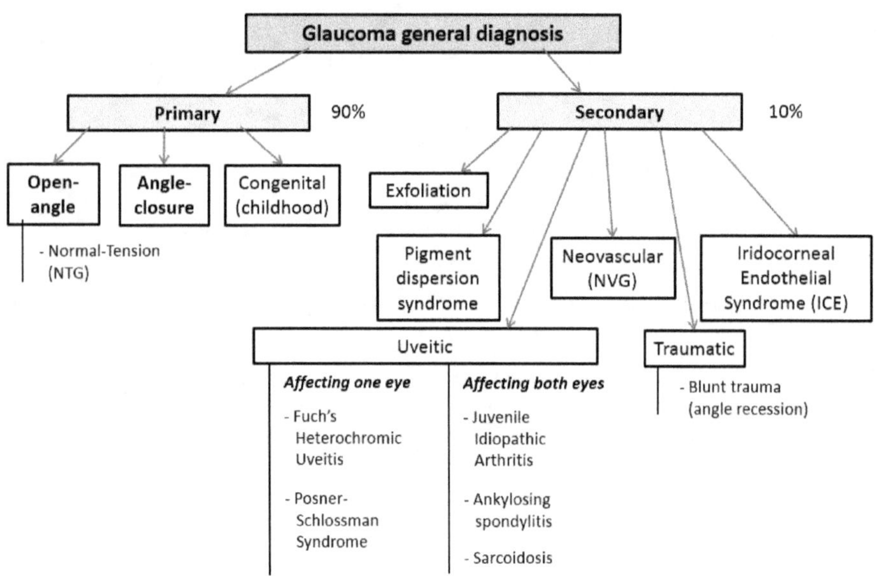

Fig. 1-1. A chart to clarify your glaucoma diagnosis. Percentages shown on the chart are approximate total occurrences in the global population, typically experienced by ophthalmologists in their clinical practices. The exact statistics might differ significantly in developed vs. developing countries, within geographic regions and individual countries, and even among ophthalmological clinics in the same city.

> Various glaucoma sub-groups require different treatments to reduce the risks of any further visual damage. *To learn your own diagnosis and to understand better your personal risks, always ask your ophthalmologist to identify your glaucoma.* Fig. 1-1 can serve as a helpful guide. Brief descriptions of each glaucoma diagnosis are presented in Appendix 2.

Your exact glaucoma diagnosis is important to know not just for yourself but also for your family. As your children and siblings face substantially increased risks for the same condition, they need to consult their own doctors for assessment and to plan their own eye care for the future.

Angle closure can be prevented with a timely relatively simple and safe laser treatment. Open-angle glaucomas cannot be prevented but if detected early, the damage to vision they can cause can be minimized.

Accurate information on your diagnosis and current treatments should be shared with your general practitioner and other medical and health support professionals, including any treatments you might be using (perhaps, on a *need-to-know basis*, with your health insurance provider). For medical experts, such knowledge might be essential to prevent unnecessary complications and drug interactions, and to minimize medication side effects and other health-related problems that you might face in the future, or to ensure that your needs are properly met.

Reaching out to the glaucoma community

You are not alone as you come to terms with your glaucoma – tens of millions of people around the world are affected. Use of internet, blogs and social media can help you to find likeminded people who could share experiences on how to overcome glaucoma-induced challenges. Often, the moving and relevant testimonials of fellow glaucoma patients might help to place your own experiences into perspective.

At the same time, be conscious that the internet also provides a platform for villains who take advantage of vulnerable people eager to find a cure; they should be avoided at all costs. The old sayings that 'if it sounds too good to be true, it most likely is', and 'buyer beware' should be applied proactively when dealing with the internet sources.

> *See information in the Appendix below on how you can identify reliable blogs dedicated to glaucoma-related issues.*

Chapter 2. Evaluations and ongoing monitoring

For diagnosed glaucoma patients, regular eye checks inevitably become a routine obligation. As stated in *Goldberg/Susanna*:

"If your treatment program is not reviewed at timely intervals or if you fail to attend for follow-up assessments or if you do not undergo some of the additional investigations (such as visual fields or optic disc measurements) as required, you are increasing the chances of failing to detect ongoing damage to your sight.

Glaucoma tends to be relentless. It seizes opportunities to destroy. It has been likened to the ocean: as you never know when the next big wave is going to come through, you never take your eyes off it. You remain vigilant. You remain alert and informed.

You and your ophthalmologist are allies against the disease. Together you need to work out a treatment strategy that is likely to work to make you safe and then to check regularly that you have been made safe.

No glaucoma patient on treatment should go for more than a year between assessments. Most glaucoma patients need three- to six-monthly reviews, depending on the severity of the damage and the apparent stability of the condition from treatment.

The milder the damage, the more effective the treatment, the longer the follow-up demonstrating stability, the longer the safe interval between visits."

> - Whether you are a large city dweller or reside in countryside far away from well-appointed medical centers, it is essential, jointly with your ophthalmologist, to devise a reasonable strategy of regular appointments. The goal of ongoing eye checks is to monitor whether deterioration in your eyesight has occurred since the last visit, and how your vision is being affected by prescribed treatments, as well as by other health and lifestyle changes that you are experiencing.
>
> - In addition, you might have to monitor the effects of the eye treatment and administered drugs on the state of your general health by seeing your medical practitioner and specialized health experts.

If you live in a developing country, arranging regular checks is usually more complicated due to the need to find time and precious resources to support your periodic travels. You might also have to overcome other non-medical difficulties, such as arranging long-distance or even international transportation, taken for granted in developed countries; common obstacles for travel if your vision is poor or you are handicapped; and universal challenges to identify qualified medical experts who are willing to see you at the exact time of your trip.

Even if you live close to a clinic, each eye check trip requires careful consideration and planning. As a rule, the more qualified your medical expert is, the more limited time you can spend together, usually just several short minutes. Hence, it is highly advisable to prepare your questions ahead, put them in writing and perhaps leave with your doctor a list of questions unanswered during the medical appointment so that you perhaps might be sent answers later with the help of the clinic staff.

For glaucoma patients, every additional testing procedure costs money, takes valuable time and effort. Sometimes, it might result in inaccurate diagnosis and needless treatment. Hence, all helpful technologies should be employed advisedly. Unnecessary medical tests do not lead to better health.

If you have been diagnosed with glaucoma, you should consider the following eye monitoring steps:

- *Schedule your regular three- to six-monthly eye examinations by an ophthalmologist.*

- Ensure that your examination always includes monitoring of IOP, a check of optic nerves, and a search for progressive damage with the appropriate use of visual fields and optic disc assessment technologies.

Measuring intraocular pressure (IOP)

Monitoring IOP during your regular visits to the ophthalmologist is an essential part of glaucoma care. IOP measurements are not trivial, often depending on a glaucoma patient's individual characteristics. For some patients it might be quite easy, whereas for the others, perhaps more challenging. Also, if you have ever had eye laser surgery, inform your ophthalmologist, as it might affect the accuracy of eye pressure measurements.

The 'gold standard' to measure the IOP is Goldmann tonometry, which uses a relatively complex procedure and device introduced by a glaucoma specialist Hans Goldmann in the 1950s. Goldmann tonometer measurement first requires instillation of drops of anesthetic and fluorescein (*i.e.*, special orange dye). Thereafter, the head of the measuring device gently touches a very small area of the front of each eye, which is being illuminated with a cobalt-blue light. There is a clear end-point that provides the eye pressure level at that moment.

Other eye pressure measurement systems are about as cumbersome; they might be somewhat less accurate and reliable. A real advance in the ability to measure IOP more frequently, preferably by the patient him/herself, would progress glaucoma treatment. Substantial progress in glaucoma care will follow when we have technology to measure IOP continuously.

For those fascinated by possible advances: ideally, IOP should be measured with the patient's eyes gently closed, including during the patient's sleep (*e.g.*, perhaps using ultrasound, or based on '*The Thing listening device*' interaction effect of electromagnetic and acoustic waves, pioneered by Léon Theremin). Alternatively, a prominent U.S. technical expert on the new glaucoma treatments, Dr. Jerrold M. Shapiro (whose post-doctoral work on glaucoma detection was done at the Boston University School of Medicine's Department of Ophthalmology, where he was Director of the Glaucoma Research Laboratory), has come up with the original idea of deploying 'elastography', currently used to detect tumors in the body. Eye's resonant frequency could be measured as a function of IOP, by 'pinging' the eye at regular intervals.

Pressure in the eye fluctuates from second to second, from day to day and from season to season – higher in winter, lower in summer. Normal living (such as drinking fluids) causes changes in your blood pressure, your heartbeat, perhaps even hormone levels. Lying down, exercising, holding your breath, playing a wind musical instrument, coughing, or pressing on the eyeball, wearing tight swimming goggles, pressing on your eyes (including with a pillow or an arm during sleep) or eye blinking, all spike your eye pressure. While healthy eyes easily handle such fluctuations, eyes with glaucoma damage might deteriorate further. According to *Goldberg/Susanna*:

"Assessing how the optic nerve fibers cope with these variations is critically important."

- The need for continual monitoring of the intraocular pressure of glaucoma sufferers is high and none of the currently commercialized monitoring technologies is optimal in terms of simplicity, flexibility, accuracy, cost and potential for self-administering the test. Perhaps people with glaucoma and glaucoma patient associations could become more proactive in their support for investigators trying to create novel technologies capable of being used at home by patients themselves. Such a mobile device should be able to monitor IOP 24 hours per day over several days, ideally not require direct contact with the patient's eyes, be cost-effective and simple to use.

- If you become aware of any new testing approaches capable of meeting these criteria, contact your local or a credible international glaucoma patient association or research foundation and support their efforts to advance IOP measurements. *See information in the Appendix below on how you can contact international or your country's glaucoma patient association, ophthalmology society or medical association that could keep you informed on the emerging scientifically proven methods of glaucoma treatment or put you in touch with the glaucoma researchers of your choice.*

Peripheral visual field testing

After IOP measurements, visual field testing ('perimetry') is the test most familiar to glaucoma patients – and one universally unpopular. It needs to be performed periodically to monitor whether your vision has deteriorated.

The *Goldberg/Susanna* book provides a detailed coverage of this important test, and the meaning of its results. A computerized device beams tiny and variably faint light points onto the inside surface of a smooth white bowl. The technician supervising the test asks you to hold your head and eyes steady and to press a button each time you think you see the light.

According to *Goldberg/Susanna*:

"At each point tested, the brightness of the projected light is varied so that the machine can measure the dimmest light you are able to see at that point. … This makes it challenging to do because the light is either just, just bright enough to be seen, or just, just too faint to be seen. You experience doubt and that is perfectly normal. To do the test most effectively, first relax, knowing that about 25% of the time, even in a totally undamaged eye, you will not see the light.

… When shown their visual field results for the first time, some patients are surprised by the damage that glaucoma has caused: they have not been aware of it. This might be dangerous: think of bicycle riding or driving or operating complex machines. Being helped to be aware of the blind spots in each eye can make a big difference as to how a patient compensates and continues to live a full and productive life safely."

Although critical to perform, for many glaucoma patients this particular test might present logistic and cost difficulties, as it often has to be scheduled with a technician right before your appointment with the ophthalmologist. Sometimes patients have to travel twice to the clinic (once for the field test, another time to see the specialist), which is especially challenging for those who live far away and for those patients with sight or mobility problems.

According to Dr. Jeffrey M. Liebmann, Clinical Professor of Ophthalmology at Columbia University School of Medicine*, certain software used by ophthalmologists is able to detect early damage of the patient's optic nerve, which otherwise is not easy to detect with an eye examination. His advice to the ophthalmologists:

"One of the best ways to avoid missing clinically meaningful progression is to take advantage of the technology that's available today. Many of the tools we use contain software that can help identify subtle changes that have occurred between exams. We're far less likely to catch these changes looking at numbers and printouts by ourselves. So, take advantage of the progression analysis software in your visual field, OCT [Optical Coherence Tomography] and other devices."

Unlike desired improvements in IOP measurements that necessitate considerable technological advances, the current state of artificial intelligence technologies enables development of smart and relatively inexpensive

---

*See *http://www.reviewofophthalmology.com/article/glaucoma-in-the-clinic-what-not-to-miss*.

gadgets capable of conducting self-tests of visual fields. If connected to a smart phone, a smart perimetry gadget should be able to provide necessary instructions and to steer a glaucoma patient through the test. It should be capable of ensuring that your head is always held properly in front of the device, your tested eye keeps looking steadily at the target light point, and that after correctly finishing the test, your smart phone would transmit its results to the physician's office, thus making unnecessary a separate trip to the clinic. In the age of self-driving cars, to achieve this relatively straightforward task requires a strong commitment from both device vendors and health professionals.

Software programs that interpret visual field results have improved greatly; currently, they can predict the likely state of your vision in the next five years based on any progression of damage over the past several years. Even though their forecasts are not yet accurate enough to guide treatment strategies on their own, in our view these predictions should be routinely provided to glaucoma patients, who need as much information as they can get to make critical decisions about their futures.

- Ask your ophthalmologist whether progression analysis of damage of your optic nerve has been performed on each of your eyes, using software analysis of your visual fields and other test equipment that the ophthalmologist used to evaluate your vision; and what its quantitative results are.

- There is definite need for a more advanced self-administering and inexpensive peripheral visual field test, which ophthalmologists, equipment vendors and glaucoma patient associations should proactively support. *See information in the Appendix below on how you can contact international or your country's glaucoma patient association, ophthalmology society or medical association that could take a proactive initiative in addressing this important issue.*

Testing central damage

According to Dr. Jeffrey M. Liebmann, glaucoma is often considered by ophthalmologists to be mainly a peripheral vision disease. Based on extensive research, he has the following advice to his colleagues:

"… glaucoma causes diffuse ganglion cell loss across the entire retina, and many patients have noticeable central loss; a patient with glaucoma can develop scotomas and other problems in the paracentral region. Loss of macular ganglion cells can lead to diminished contrast or reading ability. These problems will have visual impacts that are meaningful to the patient; in fact, they're the kind of problems that are associated with falls and fractures.

… A key part of monitoring what's happening in the patient's central vision is to simply listen to the patient. As noted above, when damage does extend to the central field it begins to affect vision in ways that patients notice. A patient may complain of difficulty reading or say that things look washed out. An astute patient may specify that his contrast sensitivity has decreased. Most ophthalmologists would assume this indicates the beginning of a cataract, but it could also indicate macular disease – or glaucoma. If a patient with known glaucoma tells you he's having increased difficulty reading, but everything else looks the same, that's probably a sign of progression even if the visual field hasn't changed. In that situation you should definitely get a 10-degree visual field."

- Ask your ophthalmologist to perform a central visual field test, if it has not yet been included in your exam.

- As with the testing of the central and peripheral visual field, there is a need for a self-administered and inexpensive test of other aspects of central vision (*e.g.*, contrast sensitivity). *See information in the Appendix below on how you can contact international or your country's glaucoma patient association, ophthalmology society or medical association that could take a proactive initiative to address this.*

Testing contrast sensitivity

Contrast sensitivity is crucially important for effective vision. Most ophthalmologists do not test it routinely. Still, it might be another way to assess whether or not your glaucoma is progressing and it might be valuable to understand how much your vision has been affected for day-to-day activities.

In their epidemiologic study*, a team of U.S. medical researchers concluded:

"The aspects of visual function that best predict the ability of a patient with glaucoma to perform activities of daily living are binocular visual acuity and contrast sensitivity."

Binocular visual acuity (*i.e.,* reading the letter chart with both eyes together) is routinely evaluated utilizing familiar charts with rows of letters that range from big ones at the top to smaller sizes at the bottom. Yet, the same study suggests that contrast sensitivity should also be tested for glaucoma patients:

"Changes in contrast sensitivity, on the other hand, occur early and provide highly valuable insight into how well patients with glaucoma are able to function. In our study, a simple, quick, low-technology method of assessing contrast sensitivity was used: asking patients to read letters of decreasing contrast. The close correlation between contrast sensitivity and the ability to perform

---

*Jesse Richman, MD; Luciano L. Lorenzana, MD; Dara Lankaranian, MD; *et al.*, Importance of Visual Acuity and Contrast Sensitivity in Patients With Glaucoma, Arch Ophthalmol. 2010;128(12):1576-1582.

activities of daily living suggests that this inexpensive test may be a highly sensitive method of assessing how glaucomatous nerve damage actually affects what people can do."

- Ask your ophthalmologist to include the test for contrast sensitivity in your periodic vision monitoring. Although loss of contrast sensitivity cannot be treated at present, it might explain to you why you are having problems at certain times with some activities.

- As with the testing of both peripheral visual field and central vision, there is a need for a self-administering and inexpensive test for contrast sensitivity. *See information in the Appendix below on how you can contact international or your country's glaucoma patient association, ophthalmology society or medical association that could take a proactive initiative in addressing this important issue.*

Measuring corneal thickness

'Ultrasound pachymetry' is the 'gold standard' procedure of evaluating the thickness of the central cornea. The normal corneal thickness at the center is on average 0.52 to 0.54 mm, depending on your sex, age and various genetic factors. If your cornea is somewhat thicker or thinner, it might affect the accuracy of IOP measurements; hence, this test has to be conducted at least once.

Newer generation pachymeters measure the corneal thickness quite accurately. Ultrasound pachymetry requires local anesthesia to maximize accuracy and your comfort.

> Ask your ophthalmologist whether ultrasound pachymetry should be performed on your eyes at least once.

Optic nerve evaluation

As written in *Goldberg/Susanna*:

"Optic nerve evaluation is an essential part of the eye examination. When necessary, it should be supplemented by photographs and scanned images from advanced technologies such as scanning laser ophthalmoscopy, scanning laser polarimetry and/or ocular coherent tomography. … Diagnosis cannot be based solely on their assessments, but to be as accurate as possible, must be made with mutually supportive information from the entire examination and assessment.

… Together with optic nerve structural assessment, visual field loss guides treatment recommendations and allows us to work out whether treatment has halted the disease or whether it is still progressing. If further damage is detected, it usually means treatment has to be made stronger to protect you. Detecting changes in the risk for more damage (higher eye pressure, for example) and assessment for progressive damage is what disease monitoring is all about."

Optic nerve evaluation includes assessment of the damage to various elements of the optic nerve with the use of complex technologies, such as disc photography, confocal scanning laser ophthalmoscopy, scanning laser polarimetry and optical coherence tomography. These are needed from time to time, the frequency, as determined by your ophthalmologist, depending on the amount of damage, the threat of that damage to your detailed focus vision and on the level of risk to your sight.

- Ensure that your ophthalmologist conducts optic nerve evaluation at your regular eye check appointments.

- Clarify with your ophthalmologist whether there is value for your eye examination being supplemented by photographs and scanned images from advanced technologies, such as scanning laser ophthalmoscopy, scanning laser polarimetry or ocular coherent tomography.

The water drinking challenge test

The 'water drinking challenge or provocative test' (WDT) is a short-cut to determine a patient's daily peak IOP, which if high, might inflict further glaucoma damage and might not be detected by once-per-visit IOP measurements. It is particularly helpful in treatment if glaucoma is advancing despite apparently 'controlled' IOP during routine visits.

As described by *Goldberg/Susanna*:

"After a couple of hours of liquid fasting, a patient either drinks 800 ml of water or 10 ml of water for each kilogram of body weight. IOP is measured before and at 15, 30, 45 and sometimes 60 minutes after drinking. IOP increases to a peak and then starts to fall. In about 87% of patients, the peak IOP after the WDT corresponds closely to the peak daily IOP. If the peak detected on treatment is above target levels for that patient, perhaps treatment should be changed so as not only to reduce IOP, but to blunt its peak levels as well.

The WDT resembles cardiac stress tests with exercise, which are widely used by cardiologists."

Evaluating ocular surface status

According to Dr. Mark B. Abelson, Clinical Professor of Ophthalmology at Harvard Medical School, and Ashley Lafond, chronic glaucoma treatment can cause, contribute to or exacerbate existing *ocular surface disease* (OSD, or a variation of it, known as '*dry eye*'):

> *"A decrease in body water in the elderly makes them susceptible to dehydration, and can play a factor in initiating or exacerbating ocular surface disease symptoms such as dryness, burning, stinging, grittiness and foreign body sensation. …*
>
> *Because both glaucoma and ocular surface disease are highly correlated with the age of the patient, ophthalmologists frequently see patients treated for glaucoma who are also exhibiting signs and symptoms of ocular surface disease … the instillation of drops can also have a detrimental effect on the ocular surface, and pulling on the lids or accidentally touching the tip of the bottle to the eye may cause irritation. … The symptoms of OSD can be severe and often debilitating, undoubtedly affecting a patient's quality of life.*
>
> *The long-term treatment plans for glaucoma with OSD can be challenging, and each patient must be considered individually, based on symptoms and ocular surface changes. … Ocular surface status should be evaluated regularly as part of a routine assessment of glaucoma patients to ensure the timely detection and treatment of pathologic signs on the ocular surface, particularly before starting a new topical therapy. …*

**See https://www.reviewofophthalmology.com/article/glaucoma-and-dry-eye-a-tough-combo.*

> *To accurately assess OSD, patients should be evaluated for ocular surface staining and tear-film breakup time prior to IOP assessments for glaucoma monitoring..."*

According to Dr. Gemma Caterina Maria Rossi from the University Eye Clinic of Pavia*, dry eye syndrome can be accurately diagnosed in glaucoma patients by several objective methods, some of which can be easily performed by the ophthalmologist in daily practice.

> If you suspect that you have dry eye problems, ask your ophthalmologist to evaluate at your regular eye check appointments the state of your ocular surface, using tear-film break-up time and Schirmer's tear test with topical anesthesia.

---

*See *https://www.reviewofophthalmology.com/article/glaucoma-and-dry-eye-a-tough-combo*.

Chapter 3. Pursuing the treatment

In this chapter, we will chart important steps to minimize further deterioration of your vision. Regrettably, today's medical practice cannot effectively heal damaged optic nerves or reverse vision loss. The most promising regenerative treatments for damaged optic nerves, such as stem cell regeneration or neuroprotection, are most likely some years away from being able to benefit people with glaucoma.

Also disappointingly, according to *Goldberg/Susanna*, even in developed countries, with their top medical and research facilities, reported blindness rates have not substantially improved for many years. This is despite many years of improvement in disease diagnosis, assessment of risk factors, eye drop medications, laser techniques and surgical approaches. Thus, a 2013 report from Sweden shows that among glaucoma patients:

"... 16.4% became blind in both eyes and 42.2% blind in one eye, of whom 20% also had severe visual damage in their fellow (better) eye... This is remarkably similar to information reported in 1965 from Olmstead County in the United States where over many years, 14% of glaucoma patients became blind in both eyes and a further 27% became blind in one eye."

Goldberg/Susanna further suggest that this situation might only be improved with ongoing scientific advances, enhanced information resources, and better communication both among eye care workers themselves and between eye workers and the community at large. Also, if you, the patient, were to be more knowledgeable and increasingly involved in your own care, they believe it could lead to better monitoring of the disease and more effective treatment, thus making a real difference in slowing down any deterioration in your vision.

This was a major motivation for us to write this handbook.

Become aware of your local or a credible international glaucoma patient association or research foundation and support their efforts to advance glaucoma treatments. Remember, with glaucoma present in your family, this is a good investment not just in your own health but also into the future for your children and grandchildren. *See information in the Appendix below on how you can contact international or your country's glaucoma patient association, ophthalmology society or medical association that could keep you informed on the emerging scientifically proven methods of glaucoma treatment or put you in touch with the glaucoma researchers of your choice.*

Controlling glaucoma

Main risk factors for onset and progression of primary glaucoma are presence of this disease in your family, your age and a high IOP. As the first two risks are not under your control, currently the only established treatment for glaucoma is to lower your eye pressure to an acceptable level. What IOP level is safe is individual for every patient and might change for a person over time.

With adequate care, for most people, glaucoma can be controlled. Your personal odds for success in glaucoma treatment mainly depend on two factors:

- The difference in IOP that treatment achieves compared with the pre-treatment.

- How fast you might be losing your vision, as measured over time.

Depending on the interaction of these two factors and results of various tests and peculiarities of your eye anatomy and functioning, different treatments can be introduced or accelerated by your ophthalmologist in order to slow or to stop glaucoma progression. The risks, costs and side effects of treatment are also taken into account to preserve your quality of life.

Reducing eye pressure

There is no 'universal' IOP level that absolutely prevents disease progression; for each patient it is different and it is also affected by age and stage of the disease.

Peak IOPs might be just as important as the overall level of IOP in your eye. Peaks can be measured with the 'water drinking challenge test' (WDT). Regular use of eye drops lowers IOP and blunts its peaks.

Goldberg/Susanna state that:

> "Determining what is the 'target' IOP for a patient is a calculated guess by the ophthalmologist depending on disease severity, life expectancy, the untreated or unsafe IOP levels, the closeness of measured vision damage to the point of fixation (which we use to read, write, recognize faces, watch TV, use computers, for example) and the presence of other contributory conditions such as central corneal thickness.

> From several large prospective clinical studies, it seems a 30% IOP reduction should prove sufficient to safeguard vision in the majority of patients with mild to moderate glaucoma. For those with more advanced damage, sometimes a 40 to 50% reduction is required. ...

> While the concept of target IOP is helpful to guide treatment strategies, it must be flexible for each patient: what might be safe when the patient is in his/her 50s, might not be safe in the same patient when he/she is in the 60s. Other conditions, such as high blood pressure being treated simultaneously, onset of diabetes, or sleep apnoea, for example, could all require a change in IOP targets. Even though the ophthalmologist is not

treating the whole patient, he/she takes into the account the health of the whole person in order to treat the eyes properly. ...

Traditionally, the glaucoma treatment approach has been to start therapy with single medications in the form of eye drops and if necessary to increase effectiveness by adding additional medicines...

If drops do not reduce your IOP as needed, there are other options such as laser therapy and a variety of incisional surgical procedures.

In some situations, your doctor may recommend surgical procedures early in your treatment, such as with far advanced glaucoma or a closed drainage system, especially if your eye pressures are very high.

Trabeculectomy [incisional surgery] remains the 'gold standard' among glaucoma surgeries. Your vision is likely to be blurred and to fluctuate after surgery, maybe even for some months. Your ophthalmologist will guide you through this carefully."

Patients' non-adherence to IOP treatment

If you, gentle reader, have made it this far in reading our book, we assume you are motivated to take your glaucoma treatment and medications seriously. It is not easy to stick to a regular routine in a busy life filled with other commitments. We hope you remain committed and succeed. Unfortunately, in doing this, many fail.

As *Goldberg/Susanna* wrote:

"Keeping the eye pressure down is what makes your vision safe, by stopping the disease process. If the treatment is used erratically and the pressures fluctuate, the disease claims a little more and then a little more of your nonrenewable vision.

… Follow the treatment plan you have worked out for you with your ophthalmologist. If you find you are not able to do so, for any reason, be sure to discuss it with him or her. …

Remember, your ophthalmologist is on your side; it is the glaucoma that is the enemy. With your ophthalmologist as your ally against the disease that is attacking you, you should be able to find a solution that works for you."

For a non-patient, it might be puzzling to understand what is the 'big deal' of putting just 3 eye drops in each eye every 12 or 24 hours for the sake of saving your vision. However, a large share of patients would never do it or, unless provided with timely information and encouragement, would stop doing it just after several weeks of halfhearted effort.

A failure to initiate prescribed treatment, to persist with it over time or to use medication properly is quite common among all patients, including those with glaucoma. Generally, the more eye drops needed each day, the less a person tends to adhere. Poor adherence to administering eye drop medication as needed means increased eye pressure and risk of progressive loss of your sight. The condition is unrelenting.

Some glaucoma patients have never before put any substances in their eyes and are reluctant or find it challenging to start doing so. But many others, who were initially motivated or who forced themselves to self-administer the drugs, might have forgotten to do so for a day or two, and then, seeing that not much has seemed to change, have become demotivated and abandon this critical process altogether.

Everybody early or later might forget to take their medications on time. If you are motivated, to prevent such a negative event, use your cell phone or computer to setup alarms (even multiple alarms if that helps), or buy a loud voice gadget, just to remind and to motivate you to instill your drops.

Medical literature shows that your knowledge about glaucoma, its treatment and having agreed goals with the ophthalmologist improves adherence. It might also mean that a person in the family who has more advanced knowledge of this disease and higher motivation might have to take on herself or himself the critical task periodically to remind the glaucoma patient to instill his/her drops and to keep appointments with the ophthalmologist.

Treatment for dry eye

Recent health research suggests that certain preservatives used in IOP-lowering eye drops might also aggravate any dry eye syndrome. Preservatives are in the bottle to suppress bacteria. According to Dr. Mark B. Abelson from Harvard Medical School, and Ashley Lafond, prescribing treatments for ocular surface disease (OSD)/dry eye to glaucoma patients should be highly individualized and take into account both conditions:

"Warm compresses on potentially affected eyelids and washing the lids with a clean washcloth, baby shampoo, or warm water using a gentle scrubbing motion, is also a useful regimen should irritation caused by bacterial contamination arise. Should a patient notice any changes in the ocular surface such as irritation, redness, swelling or itching, it's important to seek medical attention. The more time it takes for a disease to be diagnosed, the greater the likelihood the problem will become extensive, especially in cases of bacterial infection.

... Visual tasks such as reading or using a computer for an extended period of time can lead to infrequent blinking, which causes the tear film to break up more quickly, generating an unprotected ocular surface. Arid conditions such as airplane cabins can also be problematic for dry-eye patients. Advocating proper rest and hydration may be beneficial to patients with OSD symptoms. ...

There are a number of options for treating glaucoma, including medications with preservatives, preservative-free drugs and those with soft preservatives ... Many treatment options, including punctal plugs, steroids and prescription therapies, are available to patients, although most patients can manage their symptoms with over-the-counter tear substitutes to temporarily relieve the clinical signs and symptoms associated with those diseases.

Protecting the integrity of the ocular surface while treating ocular conditions like glaucoma is undoubtedly the wave of the future. Eye drops with additional ocular-surface-protective properties should become a part of an ophthalmologist's armamentarium for patients with ocular surface disorders..."

- Ask your ophthalmologist whether you should use over-the-counter tear substitutes or specialized medications to relieve dry eye syndrome, especially if you travel on an airplane (in which air is dehumidified) or to dry air destinations. As various brands of tear substitutes all try to do the same job with slightly different compositions, they might be equally helpful (or not). You could find that or one or two products might stand out for you, providing greater comfort.

- Discuss with your ophthalmologist whether you require preservative-free or 'gentle' preservatives drops, remembering that it might affect their effectiveness and anti-bacterial qualities.

- Remember to blink more often when you concentrate on visual tasks, *e.g.*, using a computer, to replenish your tear film naturally.

- Consider humidifiers in rooms where you spend significant time.

Considering your life expectancy

According to Dr. Jeffrey M. Liebmann:

"When managing a disease like glaucoma that [often] takes a long time to unfold, the amount of time left in a patient's life is an important consideration. A slow rate of progression isn't likely to lead to blindness in a patient who is 80 years old, but a patient progressing slowly at age 40 has a serious problem; he may live another 50 years. Dealing with this is a challenging aspect of glaucoma management that every clinician struggles with. How do you make a decision for a 40-year-old that might impact him 50 years later?

One mistake to avoid is under-estimating life expectancy. That's easy to do because clinicians don't always realize that life expectancy shifts the longer a person lives. At birth the average life expectancy for a man in the United States is about 75 years. But if you make it to 40, a lot of people have died along the way, so your life expectancy at that point is longer. ... This is also a consideration when deciding whether to pursue glaucoma surgery; you have to think about the ramifications down the road."

If your visual condition has not been entirely stabilized and arrested, it would be quite beneficial, jointly with your ophthalmologist and medical practitioner, to map out your treatment plan for years ahead. Typically, you would need to discuss the following critical issues, factoring them into life-changing decisions:

- How severe your visual damage is.

- How close it is to your central point of visual fixation (the sight you use to read, write, recognize faces).

- How badly affected both your eyes are.

- Realistically, what your general health is like (it gives a clue as to your likely longevity and hence how aggressive should be your eye treatment (*i.e.*, if necessary, whether it is worth to perform complex high-risk incisional surgery).

- Over time, what your response to treatment has been.

- Whether you have had progressive glaucoma damage to your vision despite past treatments. If so, what the rate of that progressive damage has been.

Exploring new treatments

Many glaucoma patients are keen to explore newer and possibly more effective treatments that could slow down or arrest further deterioration in their vision. As with many other debilitating diseases, they might read in the media or on the internet about new approaches to treat glaucoma.

It is always desirable to discuss with your ophthalmologist whether a new treatment is credible and applicable to your circumstances and state of health. On the other hand, do not attempt to treat yourself without first discussing your options with your trusted ophthalmologist.

For a patient, it is impossible to identify new treatment information by following-up countless publications and the announcements of numerous medical research and academic groups, large pharmaceutical companies, as well as startups and regulatory authorities around the globe. Patients and their family and friends that have scientific background and matching inquisitiveness, might like to look at some specialized publications that periodically compress and cover medical advances in glaucoma treatment.

Those of you that have interest in periodically updating your knowledge in new glaucoma treatments and bringing this information to the attention of your doctor, might be willing to look at least annually at the latest medical surveys of novel drugs and devices for treating glaucoma. *See information in the Appendix below on how you can find medical surveys of novel glaucoma treatments, drugs and devices.*

Chapter 4. Types of treatment

Goldberg/Susanna state:

"Traditionally, the glaucoma treatment approach has been to start therapy with single medications in the form of eye drops and if necessary to increase effectiveness by adding additional medicines. If a combination of eye drops cannot be found that is tolerated, not too inconvenient to use and strong enough to lower eye pressures to levels thought to be safe, laser treatment becomes an option. ... If none of this leads to target eye pressures, incisional surgery is the next step.

... as incisional surgery might be unpredictable in its results and carries some significant risks to vision (bleeding, infection, cataract formation, for example) it is usually reserved for a later stage in the treatment approach for most patients."

- Ask your ophthalmologist whether after the prescribed treatment the reduction in your eye pressure has been sufficient to make your vision safe – the more severe your optic nerves damage, the greater your eye pressure reduction needs to be.

- Also, ask whether the severity of the disease has progressed compared with your previous visit, as the more severe is the damage, the more careful must be the treatment.

- Do not delay starting your treatment – protection does not begin until treatment has been started.

- As much as possible, adhere to and persevere with the prescribed treatment. Work with your ophthalmologist to find ways to help you to do this.

Treatment with medications

Instilling eye drops is the only-long-term viable non-surgical treatment that lowers eye pressure. Intra-ocular pressure increases if anything blocks circulation of the watery aqueous fluid in your eye or slows down the rate of drainage.

Like all medications, anti-glaucoma drugs fall into families – some types slow down the pump while others improve drainage. New, more advanced and selective glaucoma medications, with lower side effects, have become available over the past few years and continue to appear. If you need to reduce your IOP, your ophthalmologist might prescribe combinations of medications that work by different mechanisms, where possible, combining different drugs into a single bottle for convenience and cost.

Administering eye drops

Regularly placing drops into your eyes for the rest of your life is not natural or trivial. Various glaucoma books and leaflets provide the following recommendations on properly administering your eye drops:

- Before putting drops in your eyes, wash your hands with soap and warm water, and dry them with a clean towel.

- Make sure the bottle stays clean and be careful not to let it touch any part of your eye, so that you do not transfer bacteria to the bottle's tip. Always place the bottle cap on a clean surface, such as a fresh tissue. If you have to clean the bottle because of accidental contamination, use a clean tissue.

- If the instructions say so, shake the bottle before instilling the drops.

- Start by sitting or lying down. You will increase the chances that a single drop enters the eye accurately if you lie down flat with your face up, or sit and lean back with your face up as well. Some people like to stand in front of a mirror, which helps guide them; others find standing more awkward.

- Take the cap off the bottle and have a clean tissue handy.

- Position the bottle as vertical as possible directly over your eye, close by, without touching it. While tilting your head back, pull down the lower lid of your eye with your index finger to form a pocket.

- While looking up, gently squeeze the bottle so that a single drop falls into the pocket formed by your eyelid. Close your eyes gently without squeezing.

- Eye drop medicine is quite potent. If the first drop gets inside your eye, just one drop should be sufficient, even if the bottle says "one drop or two."

- If you are not sure the first drop was instilled correctly, instill a second at that time – do not wait five minutes or more before instilling another drop as that will give you more than you need, with an increased risk of side effects. If you mistakenly instill two or more drops at the same time, the excess will spill harmlessly onto your skin (the eye can only hold the volume of one drop) where you can mop it up with the clean tissue you have to hand.

- For the drop to fully absorb into your eye, gently close your eye for 2 to 3 minutes, while gently pressing a finger on the tear drainage duct (inner corner of the eye). Try not to blink or squeeze your eyelids. The pressure on the tear duct prevents potent eye drop drugs draining to your nose from where it could enter the bloodstream and cause unwanted side effects.

- Put the cap back on the bottle.

- Using the tissue, gently clean around your eyes to remove any excess liquid.

- If you have to instill a second type of eye drop medicine, wait at least five minutes before putting it in. This will prevent the first medicine from being washed out by the second. If you have to administer both drops and ointment, use the drops first; as the ointment might form a barrier and block the drops from being absorbed.

- If you wear contact lenses, wait at least 20 minutes after instilling the drops before inserting them.

- Wash your hands again to remove any medication.

- If you forgot your drops, instill them as soon as you can and put the next lot in at the usual time.

- Store your drop bottles in a fridge before you first open them. Once you have opened a bottle, you can keep it in a cool dry place out of the fridge. Avoid keeping the bottle in your pocket, the car, or in direct sunlight where it can get overly hot.

- Eye drops should not be used after the expiry date printed on the packaging.

- Eye drops are also available in single dose disposable containers, without a preservative. Always use single dose containers just once (for both eyes together if both need them) and then discard.

- Some eye drops might irritate your eyes. Your ophthalmologist might recommend artificial tears 5 minutes before you administer the drops. Gels or ointments used at nighttime can also help soothe your eyes overnight.

- When travelling, switch your drop timings to the place where you happen to be, even if the interval between drops is temporarily increased or decreased.

These are general recommendations that might have to be modified for your own use. Discuss with your ophthalmologist or pharmacist which procedures and medicines might suit you better, which of many possible side effects might result from such procedures and medicines and how you might reduce these side effects on your body and wellbeing. Always notify your family doctor of the types of glaucoma drugs taken and read information on the side effects given with the bottle by your pharmacist.

We all might forget to take required medicines on time. Although eye drops do not have to be used at exactly the same time each day, using a simple alarm might help you to remember. With your ophthalmologist, select a convenient daily time slot that it is easier for you to remember. *Goldberg/Susanna* recommend linking eye drops with landmarks in your day, such as after waking, when shaving, with breakfast or dinner, when brushing teeth or when retiring to bed. Do whatever works best for you.

According to Dr. Michael Steiner, an eye surgeon from Sydney, Australia (see *https://www.nps.org.au/australian-prescriber/articles/on-the-correct-use-of-eye-drops*):

"… The current policy is that once eye drops have been opened they should be disposed of after 28 days. This is based on research from earlier times when drops were dispensed in glass bottles with glass pipettes, and many eye drops did not contain preservatives. To my knowledge none of this research is current, using modern dropper-type bottles. This policy seems a terrible waste and causes increased expense to the patients and the health system.

Although evidence is needed to support the practice, some ophthalmologists allow patients who are using drops regularly to keep the bottle for up to two months (although most of them run out after about six weeks)."

For many glaucoma patients, especially the more elderly, with poorer eyesight or motor coordination, tremor or arthritis, their ability to self-administer eye drops is quite limited. Your ophthalmologist might not appreciate you are having physical difficulties with self-instillation unless you volunteer this information.

Some online stores, glaucoma associations and local pharmacies around the world sell eye drop-dispensing devices that can help you get drops in your eyes with more precision. These dispensing devices might hold the eye open and direct the drop to the eyelid pocket and not out of the eye, the dosage is easier to control and the bottle does not touch the eye. Although by no means ideal and sometimes difficult to buy in your own country, if available and suitable for you and for the exact bottle(s) you are using, they might improve the accuracy of putting drops in your eyes, especially eyes with low vision. Overall, such devices could improve patient adherence and reduce reliance on others to administer drops. Not less important, they might somewhat reduce wasting expensive eye drop medicine and hence your need to refill the prescription quite so often.

Unfortunately, there is no ideal eye drop-dispensing device compatible with all eye drop bottles. You might need to shop around until you find a device that suits your eye anatomy and is appropriate for the bottles with drops that you might use at a given time.

- There are numerous text and graphics instructions and videos on the internet on eye drop instillation. *See information in the Appendix below on how you can find tips and videos for administering eye drops that could better fit your individual needs.*

- Eye drop dispensing devices could be used by patients with limited ability to self-administer eye drops. *See information in the Appendix below on how you can find eye drop dispensing devices in your country or in online stores.*

- As 3D-printing in medical applications has been proliferating around the world, it would be highly beneficial if some passionate volunteers could produce open source, collaborative designs of anti-blinking and precise drop dispensing devices. Such drawings should be adjustable to any individual's eye anatomy. The output devices should be compatible with various eye drop bottles and should help someone to squeeze the bottle with relative ease in order to instill the drops accurately on the first attempt. Such a device should last and be easy to clean. That would provide glaucoma patients in the developed and developing countries alike, their caregivers, relatives and friends, with inexpensive ways to print easily customizable eye drop dispensers.

Non-invasive laser glaucoma procedures

Laser trabeculoplasty is a non-invasive procedure; it might be recommended as first-line therapy to reduce IOP or used if medications fail to lower eye pressures sufficiently (as an add-on to ongoing drops) or cause unacceptable side effects (as a replacement for discontinued drops). It has been shown to be safe and might offer long lasting benefits. It might be an effective substitute for drops or useful to add to one or more medications to accelerate treatment; complications are few, although rarely the IOP might rise rather than fall. It is performed with just a few drops of anesthetic.

Although exact mechanisms of action for this laser procedure are not well understood, it is believed that it improves outflow of the aqueous fluid, thus reducing IOP. Laser applications onto the cells of the drain might stimulate release of locally active hormones within the drain tissues, thereby lowering resistance to outflow, and thus dropping IOP. For some treatments, pressure lowering has also been observed on the untreated eye, which suggests that a biological effect is taking place in the human body.

The biochemical changes that positively affect the flow and reduce the pressure might take several weeks to become fully effective and might provide a benefit for several years. Benefit might be less for some kinds of glaucoma and for patients who are younger.

In laser peripheral iridotomy, laser energy vaporizes a small hole through the iris tissue, creating a by-pass for aqueous fluid to the drain, allowing it to open wider for those with angle-closure.

As with all treatments, non-invasive glaucoma procedures are not a cure and your IOP might unexpectedly rise again. If that happens, a repeated non-invasive procedure could help once more. The important point to remember is that at present glaucoma cannot be cured – it can be controlled, but must always be monitored. If it jumps out of control, most likely, it will not give you any warning.

Minimally invasive glaucoma procedures

The goal of these relatively new procedures is to provide less invasive ways to reduce eye pressure compared with conventional drainage surgery. Their numbers are growing – since June 2012 the U.S. Food and Drug Administration (FDA) has approved several micro-implantable devices. They mainly benefit patients with milder to moderate glaucoma, or who are intolerant of or non-compliant with eye pressure lowering drops and non-responsive to the non-invasive laser procedure.

All patients are subjected to a pre-operative comprehensive eye and general health exams, to ensure that a prescribed procedure is indeed suitable for them. Not all these procedures are 'right' for everyone.

These micro-procedures are performed under the microscope with tiny incisions, which are much less intrusive and hence generally safer than full surgery. As well, the implantable tubes and devices are small.

Such procedures might be combined with cataract surgery, which extends that surgery slightly, with minimal additional inconvenience to the patient. They are designed to be quick, require few steps, performed by suitably trained ophthalmologists. However, cataract surgery on its own might also reduce IOP even without a glaucoma add-on procedure.

According to a publication of the American Academy of Ophthalmology*:

"Clinical trials have shown there to be a significant decrease in IOP over periods of up to 24 months along with a significant decrease in medication usage."

Although resulting reductions in IOP are typically smaller than for conventional incisional surgery, their risks and side effects, in particular of infection and scarring, are lower and post operational recovery times faster. Patients have a more rapid visual recovery than with the traditional full surgery. If the IOP has not been substantially reduced with a minimally invasive glaucoma procedure, full incisional surgery remains possible.

Fortunately, the variety of minimally invasive glaucoma procedures and devices continues to increase, with some more likely to lower IOP more effectively than others. Also, possible complications are different for various procedures.

---

*See   *http://eyewiki.aao.org/Microinvasive_Glaucoma_Surgery_(MIGS)*.

- However minimally invasive, every operation has its own set of risks and potential side effects. As medical practice is as much art as it is science, the outcome of any operation depends on the experience and diligence of the surgeon. Always discuss with your ophthalmologist before the operation its potential best and worst outcomes and risk/benefit ratio for you as an individual. Be sure you are comfortable with what has been proposed for you and ask about other possibilities.

- Consider obtaining a second qualified medical opinion on whether your prescribed operation is necessary beyond any doubt. Always understand possible benefits and balance them against potential risks.

Incisional surgery

A particular kind of conventional incisional surgery to reduce IOP called '*trabeculectomy*' has evolved steadily since first popularized in the late 1960s. It is usually necessary if IOP is very high, while visual damage is severe and progresses despite other treatments (especially when approaching the center of the visual field); that is, if the risk of *not* operating exceeds the risk of operating. This surgery requires meticulous technique and careful post-operative supervision.

Incisional surgery creates a drainage channel out of the eye for the aqueous fluid back to the blood stream. During and for the first four weeks after the operation, the patient needs arduous care, and must use certain medicines to reduce inflammation. Otherwise, this surgery could result in the creation of scar tissue that would seal the new artificial channel. As the newly formed channel is 'unnatural', the body tries to heal it but, while healing, it seals it, so that IOP increases once again. During this critical time, vision might fluctuate and be blurry.

Another post-operation challenge is to keep the IOP within an optimal range. Both too low and too high eye pressures negatively affect vision and might require additional interventions.

If the operation has been successful, IOP might be stably controlled for many years at target levels, offering maximal visual safety. As with many complex operations, glaucoma surgery outcomes are not entirely predictable and carry various complications (such as raised IOP, blurred vision, astigmatism), and risks of side effects (bleeding, infections and cataract formation or acceleration).

Successful incisional surgery typically results in a raised 'blister' under the upper eyelid, called the 'bleb'. This artificial drainage channel-outflow pathway might become too big and thus require another (usually relatively minor) surgery, to correct it.

Every treatment might have complications. *Goldberg/ Susanna* wrote that:

> "If you've had a glaucoma operation and you develop an infection, seek help immediately.
>
> Clues that you might have an infection include an eye that is red and irritable, especially with a yellowy pus discharge or with eyelid stickiness, particularly when you awake in the mornings."

Because of these possible complications and relative unpredictability, incisional surgery is only considered if the risk of not doing the operation exceeds the risk of doing it. Risk of scarring and failure to control the IOP increases if the eye has undergone similar surgery previously.

Glaucoma and cataract

Goldberg/Susanna state that:

"As both glaucoma and cataract increase in frequency as people age, they are often found together. Furthermore, both long-term anti-glaucoma medications … and glaucoma (or other) eye surgery can produce or accelerate cataract formation. …

Because the results of modern cataract surgery are so good, the chances of success are so high (usually about 95-97%) and the recovery is so predictable for otherwise-normal eyes, cataract surgery has become the most common operation of any kind performed in many countries. However, as it is not 100% safe and it is not 100% free from possible problems, it is usually advised only when visual problems justify the small risk of something unwanted happening.

In eyes with glaucoma and glaucoma damage to the vision (or any other eye problems, like macular degeneration or diabetic eye disease, for example), successful cataract surgery can only restore the sight to the level permitted by the other eye diseases. Therefore, it is important to have realistic expectations from any surgical interventions."

If both cataract and glaucoma surgeries are necessary, they might be combined into one operation. Alternatively, the ophthalmologist might recommend cataract surgery first, in the hope it could benefit pressure control enough to allow glaucoma surgery to be postponed or even deferred indefinitely. Preferably, glaucoma surgery should not be scheduled before planned cataract surgery, as the subsequent cataract surgery can induce scarring in a functioning incisional surgery, spoiling its performance.

Chapter 5. Glaucoma and your health and lifestyle

As with any other severe disease, you have to take into account potential effects of glaucoma when dealing with other health issues or when considering work, travel, sport, fitness and recreational activities.

Glaucoma and general health

- According to a survey by U.S. optometrists Tammy P. Than and Erin B. Hardie*, many common medications can exacerbate existing glaucoma by increasing IOP in glaucoma patients, although such adverse effects are relatively rare. Older glaucoma patients are more likely to use multiple medications for chronic conditions, while their general health is less robust; hence, they are at increased risk for adverse drug effects.

- In particular, if you are a glaucoma patient or a child or sibling of a glaucoma patient, and need to use steroids of any kind (tablets, inhaled sprays, creams, injections, and especially eye drops), do not overuse them; use them only when you have to, no more and no less. Remember to tell all the doctors looking

*See *https://www.reviewofoptometry.com/ce/meds-that-dont-mix-with-glaucoma-patients*.

after you that you are taking steroids and that you or your direct relatives have glaucoma. While steroids can increase IOP in some healthy people, they can do so more frequently and more quickly in patients with glaucoma.

- An acute angle-closure crisis might occur when internal eye structures are blocked, which leads to a spike in IOP and damage to the optic nerve. Such an attack could be triggered by stress or could suddenly occur when awake in a dark room (*e.g.,* in a movie theater). Taking medications that dilate the pupil (*i.e.,* certain antidepressants, treatments for common cold, antihistamines and anti-nausea drugs) could also lead to an attack. An acute attack might be stopped by IOP reducing drops or by laser or surgical means. According to Gary Heiting, OD*:

"Acute angle-closure (closed-angle or narrow-angle) glaucoma produces symptoms such as eye pain, headaches, [colored rings] around lights, dilated pupils, vision loss, red eyes, nausea and vomiting.

These signs may last for hours or until the IOP is reduced. With each narrow-angle glaucoma attack, part of your peripheral vision may be lost.

Acute angle-closure glaucoma is a medical emergency. If the high eye pressure is not reduced within hours, it can cause permanent vision loss. Anyone who experiences these symptoms should

---

*See *http://www.allaboutvision.com/conditions/narrow-angle-glaucoma.htm*.

contact an ophthalmologist immediately or go to a hospital emergency room."

- Discuss with your ophthalmologist, medical practitioner, and other medical and health support specialists, such as cardiologist, endocrinologist, surgeon, dentist and pharmacist, whether prescribed medications or various medical treatments might have side effects on the IOP and the state of your vision.

- Carefully read instructions attached to each medication that you have been prescribed, to find out whether a particular drug might be unsafe for glaucoma patients.

- In cases of eye pain, headaches, colored rings around lights, dilated pupils, vision loss, red eyes, nausea and vomiting, immediately contact your ophthalmologist or go to a hospital emergency room.

- Various books and scientific articles help to determine whether a particular medication, vitamins, herbal and nutritional supplement or other chemical might further aggravate glaucoma. *See information in the Appendix below on how you can search for such published sources.*

Glaucoma and eyeglasses

Glaucoma patients often become sensitive to light and glare; this might indicate developing cataracts or other types of vision loss. Light sensitivity could be further aggravated by the application of eye drops. Hence, glaucoma patients should wear sunglasses when they are subjected to bright light, to get protection from harmful ultraviolet (UV) rays.

The American Academy of Ophthalmology recommends using sunglasses that block 99 or 100% of UV light or that are labeled for UV absorption 'up to 400 nm'. Polarized lenses reduce reflected glare; hence, they might be particularly useful for driving and water-related sports, such as fishing.

A medium dark lens is good for day-to-day activities, driving and playing sports. If you are out in the sun, especially with snow, water or other very bright conditions, choose darker lenses, which should not allow you to see your eyes in a mirror.

Wraparound glasses are shaped to keep light from shining into your eyes from the sides, as well as from the front. Large-framed wraparound sunglasses can protect your eyes better from light reaching you at all angles.

Effect of glaucoma on your lifestyle

As with other potentially debilitating diseases, glaucoma might affect daily routines and long-term lifestyle decisions. Perhaps suddenly, choices range from the mundane – *i.e.,* when selecting the time you and your spouse could travel to a store after placing drops into your eyes; to the more strategic – such as buying a house in a retirement community close to a specialized medical center that would accept you as a glaucoma patient, or considering whether your next car should have self-driving functions.

Various medical and epidemiological studies have shown that visual acuity worsens in the later stages of glaucoma. At that stage, affected patients often experience significant difficulties when performing routine daily tasks. In particular, walking speed might be slower; they might bump into more objects, and have a slower reading speed. They might also have problems with detecting motion, navigating obstacles, and finding objects.

According to *Goldberg/Susanna*:

"Aerobic exercises (swimming, jogging, cycling, rowing) for at least 30 minutes three times weekly can help to reduce your eye pressures. Such activities also improve your blood pressure and cholesterol, your weight control and your sugar metabolism, all of which help to keep the little blood vessels at the back of your eyes around your optic nerves healthier.

Avoid head-down yoga-type positions as this increases eye pressure, and musicians who play wind instruments might need to discuss this with their ophthalmologist. All these activities can increase eye pressure. They also increase pressure around the brain, however, which might protect the optic nerves from the effects of the raised eye pressures, so we do not know whether or not people need to consider stopping such activities.

If you swim with goggles, ensure they are large enough to sit against the bones of your face and NOT against your eyeballs; if goggles push against the eyes, they increase their pressure, sometimes dramatically.

Another possible cause of high eye pressure is tying a necktie too tightly. This might hinder the flow of blood in the neck veins returning blood from the head, brain and eyes to the heart and as the eyes drain into these veins (they are 'upstream' from them), any rise in vein pressure will increase eye pressure. So avoid wearing shirts or blouses whose collars are too tight for you or tying neckties too tightly.

When you are sleeping or simply lying down, you are horizontal. Lying supine (on your back, facing the ceiling) increases eye pressure because the eyes become level with the heart; compare this with sitting or standing positions where gravity helps blood flow down to the heart and lowers the pressure in the veins of the head, into which the eyes are draining. This is normal and cannot be avoided. However, it is made worse if you lie prone (chest downwards) with your head turned to one side, because it is easy for your eyes to press against the pillows and bedding. Pressure on the eyeball increases IOP and although the pressure slowly equalizes, there is a period when it could be high.

Ensure therefore that your eyes are not making contact with anything when you sleep and if it is comfortable for you to do so, consider elevating the head of the bed slightly. Propping yourself up on more cushions does not seem to lower eye pressures as much as raising the head of the bed.

Smoking not only can increase eye pressure, but it can lead to damage to the vital small blood vessels around the optic nerves; damage to these blood vessels can make them more vulnerable to glaucoma damage. Marijuana (tetrahydrocannabinol or THC) decreases eye pressures, but only when used at the level that also affects mental function. Unfortunately, the active ingredients in delta-9 THC that lower IOP have not been able so far to be separated from their effects on mood and thinking, despite much effort!"

A range of 'vision rehabilitation' tools can help patients with advanced glaucoma to reduce the negative effects of low vision. In particular, numerous specialized devices, computer programs, occupational therapy, as well as physical, mobility and home skills training, could offer a real and lasting improvement for low vision glaucoma patients, greatly enhancing their quality of life. You might also benefit from vision rehabilitation services and consultants who train low vision persons in the use of such tools. Together with your ophthalmologist, seek out such help before it becomes a critical necessity.

> Various government organizations, non-for-profit associations, private companies and stores provide low vision rehabilitation training and tools. *See information in the Appendix below on how you can search for such organizations.*

Glaucoma and your food

Although your choice of food is unlikely to cure glaucoma, it could contribute to your overall health and, possibly, help to support the state of your vision.

Thus, according to a study conducted by a team of medical researchers from Harvard University*, a diet high in fruits and vegetables might reduce the risk of exfoliation syndrome, which is the most common cause of secondary open angle glaucoma. The study has shown that the risk for glaucoma reduces with the increase in intake of fruits and vegetables.

There are also some indications that beets are especially beneficial for exfoliation glaucoma patients.

> - As food choices highly depend on your individual and cultural preferences, and because various types of glaucoma might be affected by food quite differently, it is worth to discuss your diet with your ophthalmologist, medical practitioner and nutritional experts.
>
> - *See information in the Appendix below on how you can search for information on the effect of diet on particular types of glaucoma.*

---

*See   http://jamanetwork.com/journals/jamaophthalmology/fullarticle/1853492.

Planning for a medical emergency

Even though each of us should hope for a long, productive and independent life, some glaucoma patients might suddenly experience substantial worsening or loss of vision. Most of us much prefer to postpone or avoid addressing unpleasant imaginary choices. However, you owe it to yourself and to the people that depend on you or that you care about, to address such issues before they might actually happen. Also, it might be much easier for your family and friends to assist you in case you are incapacitated, if they knew your wishes.

- For every person, there are numerous unique legal, business, monetary, cultural and religious factors that define their actions in case they are incapacitated.

- Discuss with your lawyer or banker and with trusted family members or friends how to structure critical legal documents: your will, healthcare directive and appointment of a healthcare agent, enduring power of attorney, and a living trust.

- Various government, legal and banking guides, books and articles could help you to determine how to assemble your personal health, legal and financial data and structure essential documents that your family and friends should read in case of a personal emergency. *See information in the Appendix below on how you can search for such published sources.*

- Ensure that persons you trust know how to get such documents in an emergency, are empowered to make necessary payments on your behalf and to assemble required caregiver arrangements.

Appendix 1. Glaucoma diagnosis

Table 1-1. Glaucoma general diagnosis

Glaucoma sub-type	Description	Share of population affected	Forecast
Glaucoma	The optic nerve has been damaged.	• 0.5% at the age of 40; • 2% of over 40 years old; • 8% of 80 year olds.	Cannot be generalized; see specific diagnoses below.
Primary	Optic nerve damage occurs without any detectable cause.	90% of glaucomas.	Cannot be generalized; see specific diagnoses below.

Glaucoma sub-type	Description	Share of population affected	Forecast
Secondary	Optic nerve damage occurs due to external or internal conditions, *i.e.*, injuries, prolonged use of steroid medication, eye inflammation, or problems with the focusing lens or cornea.	10% of glaucomas.	Better outlook if cause can be identified and treated; otherwise treatment success depends on effective glaucoma control.

Table 1-2: **Primary glaucoma diagnosis**

Glaucoma sub-type	Description	Share of population affected	Forecast
Open-angle	Glaucoma occurs without any detectable cause. Normal-tension glaucoma (NTG), also called low-tension or normal-pressure glaucoma is a sub-type of primary open-angle glaucoma. The optic nerve is damaged even though the eye pressure is not very high (usually between 12-20 mm Hg). The cause of damage is usually unknown. At higher risk for NTG are people: • with a family history of normal-tension glaucoma; • of Japanese/Korean ancestry; • with a history of systemic heart disease.	75% of total glaucomas. More common in people with African ancestry.	Open-angle glaucoma is responsible for 50% of glaucoma visual disability For NTG, because IOP is 'normal', diagnosis is often confirmed later than for high-IOP glaucomas. This emphasizes the importance of optic nerve evaluation at all treatment stages.

Glaucoma sub-type	Description	Share of population affected	Forecast
Angle-closure	Glaucoma usually occurs due to external or internal conditions, *i.e.*, injuries, use of decongestants for coughs and colds, treatments for bladder problems, antidepressants, eye inflammation, or problems with the focusing lens or cornea. For some populations it is facilitated by the inherited anatomic elements of the individual's eye and further deteriorates with aging. Usually affect both eyes. If of sudden onset, might cause severe pain, headaches, nausea and vomiting, blurring of vision, sensations of rainbow rings around lights. If untreated, could destroy sight in days. Almost all oral medications contraindicated in glaucoma are linked to this type of glaucoma. Most commonly chronic and asymptomatic.	25% of total glaucomas. Affects women more than men. More common in Chinese, Indian, other Asian and Inuit populations.	Responsible for 50% of glaucoma visual disability, because its diagnosis is often missed, even more than for the open-angle glaucoma.

Glaucoma sub-type	Description	Share of population affected	Forecast
Congenital (childhood)	Occurs in babies when there is incorrect or incomplete development of the eye's drainage canals during the prenatal period.	This relatively rare condition is quite often inherited. Very small percentage of diagnosed glaucomas.	Microsurgery can correct the structural defects. Results often better when uncomplicated by other abnormalities.

Table 1-3: Open-angle glaucoma sub-diagnosis

Glaucoma sub-type	Description	Share of population affected	Forecast
Exfoliative, also called pseudoexfoliative	LOXL-1 gene abnormality has been associated with this particular condition. Abnormal material that looks like microscopic dandruff is released in the eye where it damages the drain and rubs on the iris, releasing its pigment granules into the watery fluid, further blocking drain channels and raising eye pressure, often rapidly and severely. This in turn might damage the optic nerve.	More common in older people and certain ethnic groups, including: Russian Jews; people from the Nordic countries; Greeks and others Mediterranean populations; Indians.	Tends to be a more aggressive form of glaucoma, but the underlying exfoliation syndrome might be found with no evidence of glaucoma.

Table 1-4: **Secondary glaucoma diagnosis**

Glaucoma sub-type	Description	Share of population affected	Forecast
Pigmentary dispersion	Pigment granules from the back of the iris are dislodged by rubbing, float with the aqueous fluid, blocking and damaging the drainage channel. The eye pressure rises. This in turn might damage the optic nerve. Affects most commonly slightly shortsighted men in their 20s-30s.	Although this is a relatively uncommon condition, it is more common among younger people, mostly men.	As with the underlying exfoliation syndrome, pigmentary dispersion can occur without glaucoma. Usually treated like primary open-angle glaucoma, with some differences in the type of laser procedure performed in the affected eye.

Glaucoma sub-type	Description	Share of population affected	Forecast
Traumatic	Mostly caused by a blunt injury to the eye and occasionally injuries that penetrate the eye; occurs either immediately after an injury or years later (called angle-recession glaucoma). Examples include a blow to the eye from sportsrelated injuries (in baseball, boxing, squash). Angle recession highlights the damage done to the drainage canals in the eye with pressure increases sometimes many years after the injury. Other conditions, such as severe nearsightedness, previous injury, infection or prior surgery might also contribute.	The greater the extent of injury (seen as angle recession), the higher the risk. Glaucoma might occur up to 30 years later.	Treated similarly to a more aggressive form of primary open-angle glaucoma. If you have had an eye injury, you should have regular checks by an ophthalmologist for the rest of your life, to ensure that any subsequent glaucoma is detected early and efficient treatment offered to safeguard your vision.

Glaucoma sub-type	Description	Share of population affected	Forecast
Neovascular (NVG), also called new vessel, hemorrhagic, thrombotic, congestive, rubeotic, and diabetic hemorrhagic	NVG diagnosis usually covers numerous blinding diseases, most commonly associated with retinal vein blockage or diabetic eye disease.	The better controlled a person's diabetes and the more efficient the treatment after a retinal vein obstruction, the less likely is NVG to develop.	Treatment starts with identification and correction of the cause. Newer medications and laser approaches have revolutionized treatment, but outlook for visual recovery depends on the underlying cause, how much visual damage it has caused and how amenable it is to treatment.
Irido corneal endothelial syndrome (ICE)	ICE is a rare form of glaucoma, usually found in only one eye. Symptoms include hazy vision upon awakening and the appearance of colored rings around lights.	Rare. Cause unknown.	ICE is difficult to treat; it causes visual damage through corneal decompensation, as well as glaucoma.

Glaucoma sub-type	Description	Share of population affected	Forecast
Uveitic	Uveitic glaucoma diagnosis usually covers numerous inflammation disorders (*e.g.*, sarcoidosis, tuberculosis, toxoplasmosis and various viruses) that increase eye pressure; some affect only one eye: • Fuchs' Heterochromic Iridocyclitis; • Posner-Schlossman Syndrome; • Herpetic uveitis. • Other forms can affect both eyes: • Juvenile idiopathic arthritis; • Ankylosing spondylitis; • Sarcoidosis.	20% of patients with ocular inflammatory disorders (uveitis).	With modern treatments focusing on the root cause of inflammation, as well as controlling the eye pressure, many patients are able to maintain excellent vision.

Appendix 2. Suggested information searches

We do not cite any particular published reviews of the support equipment for visually impaired, especially computer-based, or refer you to any specific brands, partly because they rapidly become obsolete. Another reason for you to search for the most recent information is that your needs from such equipment could be quite distinct, and hence it might require individual customization, which is usually also rapidly dates.

Instead, to obtain objective and up-to-date equipment or treatment recommendations, you might consider **consulting your trusted health practitioner or conducting internet searches** using your favorite search engine, as the need arises.

For introduction: Search examples

Text to Speech (TTS) software

- Text to Speech (TTS) software was first developed to aid the visually impaired, by converting digital text (*i.e.,* retrieved on internet or a word processor file) into spoken voice. To conduct an internet search for the latest TTS software, you can use the following search statement:

text to speech software reviews

A large share of TTS is being distributed on the internet for 'free' or at low cost.

Gadgets for visually impaired

- To conduct internet search for the latest computerized gadgets for visually impaired, use the following search statement:

  text to speech blind

  This search would likely result in comparative surveys or general descriptions of the professional products for the blind, both online software and standalone devices, which are often not that cheap.

Computerized language translation

- To identify suitable systems and services for computerized language translation, search for:

  best translation software

- If you need to search for a specific or uncommon translation language service, with the specialized scientific vocabulary, search instead for:

  english to mongolian medical text translation

  that is, if you are interested in translating this book on the fly to the Mongolian language.

For Chapter 1 - Coming to terms: First steps
Identifying genetic testing services

* To conduct internet search, you can use the following search statement:
  medical genetic testing services review

* Note that at present, commercial genetic testing services mostly serve certain countries or, due to the regulatory restrictions, just conduct ancestry genetic tests. If such online service is unavailable in your locality, try to identify a locally licensed medical laboratory that provides genetics services as a part of health counseling, in which case search for:
  [country] medical genetic testing
  i.e., if you are located in Australia, search for:
  australia medical genetic testing

Finding target association's coordinates

* Search for:
  [country] glaucoma association
  i.e., if you are located in the UK, search for:
  UK glaucoma association

* If you are located in a non-English speaking country, translate the above search into the local language.

* If you cannot find a glaucoma society at your country or state, access Web site of the World Glaucoma Patient Association (*http://worldgpa.org*). They will be

able to guide you to your national patient association.

- Consider the UK International Glaucoma Association (IGA, *glaucoma-association.com*), Glaucoma Australia (*glaucoma.org.au*), the Glaucoma Foundation in New York (*glaucomafoundation.org*) or the Glaucoma Research Foundation in San Francisco (*glaucoma.org*) whose missions are to raise awareness of glaucoma, promote research related to early diagnosis and treatment, and to provide support to patients and caregivers. They might be able to refer you to a local glaucoma group or you might consider a donation to a research fund supported or recommended by the IGA.

- Alternatively, you might search for:
    [country] ophthalmology society
  or to:
    [country] medical association
  or to:
    [country] glaucoma patient association
  whose staff would likely refer you to the credible academics and professionals involved in glaucoma research and treatment that might need your support or put you in touch with a reputable ophthalmologist in a country of your choice.

Finding foreign country's trade representatives

- Search for:
    [target country's] (embassies OR consulates) in [your country]

i.e., if you are located in the USA, search for:
> *indian (embassies OR consulates) in the USA*

Note that for obtaining effective results in some search engines, in the above statement OR operator has to be capitalized and rounded brackets have to be placed exactly as shown.

- If you are located in a non-English speaking country, translate the above search into the local language.

- After identifying a nearby consulate or embassy for your target country, contact its commercial section and ask their trade representative to put you in touch with their country's leading medical clinics specializing in treating eye diseases.

Finding blogs dedicated to glaucoma-related issues

- Search for:
> *glaucoma blog*

For Chapter 3 - Pursuing the treatment

Finding tips for administering eye drops

- To conduct internet search, you can use the following search statement:

  handling eye drops

Finding videos for administering eye drops

- Search for:

  eye drops video

Finding eye drop dispenser devices

- Search for:

  [country] eye drops aids

  i.e., if you are located in the India, search for:

  india eye drops aids

Exploring new treatments

- Search for:

  novel glaucoma IOP therapy drugs devices

For Chapter 5 - Glaucoma and your health and lifestyle

Identifying general publications on side effects of medication, vitamins and herbal supplement or other chemical for glaucoma patients

- To conduct internet search, use the following search statement:

  glaucoma medications to avoid

Searching for side effects of a particular substance on glaucoma patients

- Search for:

  [substance] glaucoma side effects

  i.e., if you are searching for side effects of steroid prednisone, search for:

  prednisone side effects glaucoma

Identifying organizations that provide vision rehabilitation training

- Search for:

  [country] low vision rehabilitation training

  i.e., if you are located in the New Zealand, search for:

  new zealand low vision rehabilitation training

Searching for stores selling low vision rehabilitation tools

- Search for:
    [city, country] stores for visually impaired
  i.e., if you are located in Toronto, Canada, search for:
    toronto stores for visually impaired

Searching for information on the effect of diet on particular types of glaucoma

- Search for:
    [type of glaucoma] diet
  or just:
    glaucoma diet

Identifying government, legal and banking guides, books and articles, which could help you to determine how to structure documents that your family and friends should read in case of a personal emergency

- To conduct internet search, use the following search statement:
    affairs in order checklist

Index of recommended search terms

Walking   93
Water Drinking challenge Test (WDT)   52, 58
Wind instruments   93

Yoga   93, 94

www.ingramcontent.com/pod-product-compliance
Lightning Source LLC
LaVergne TN
LVHW011020200726
843509LV00011B/1164